REGENESIS: LIVING THE WAY THE CREATOR
INTENDED

Published by Sanear Corporation Publishing
301 E John St, Ste 973
Matthews, NC 28106

ReGenesis: Living the Way the Creator Intended
LC Control Number: 2017949986
ISBN-10: 0-692-92450-7
ISBN-13: 978-0-692-92450-1

Sanear Corporation Publishing
301 E John St, Suite 973
Matthews, NC 28106
jgsmith@sanearcorp.com

Information in this book is intended to help readers make
informed decisions about their health and the health of
family. Some information contained in this book is
based on analysis and conclusions of the author. Please
consult your doctor for specific medical advice.

Book and Cover Design by James G. Smith

Printed in the United States of America

First Edition

REGENESIS:
LIVING THE WAY
THE CREATOR INTENDED

POWERFUL WAYS TO NATURALLY
RESTORE AND ENHANCE YOUR HEALTH

By James G. Smith

Sanear Corporation Publishing

Table of Contents

REGENESIS:
LIVING THE WAY
THE CREATOR INTENDED

Powerful Ways to Naturally Restore and
Enhance Your Health

INTRODUCTION

"...You shall eat the herb
of the field."

NKJV Genesis: 3:18
Said the Lord our GOD, the Creator of all things

How can you live a longer healthier life? The creator gave us the directive during the earliest days of human existence, which involves something most people do daily. In addition, both doctors and scientists agree - the key to physical and mental health, as well as, longevity lies in what you eat and daily physical activity.

The reason I wrote this book is personal. About 5 years ago, I experienced a wake-up call, as a result of my annual physical. I worked out 2 to 3 times weekly, lifting weights and running or playing basketball. So, my mindset was that I'll get great feedback from my doctor and my numbers would be perfect - well they weren't. I was a ticking time bomb and didn't know it. My report came back indicating that I was pre-hypertensive and pre-diabetic, poised for potential heart disease and diabetes. The doctor said he wanted to see me again in 3 months. Wow, it didn't make any sense, but as I examined my lifestyle, it made perfect sense.

Well, I worked at a desk job, sitting for 6 to 8 hours daily. Second, I had 16 ounces of sweet tea with lunch daily – yes, I live in the south. Finally, I had delicious chocolate or oatmeal cookies with green tea after dinner nightly. After, the scary medical report, I decided to make a radical life change. I already knew what to do, but didn't practice it. So, I completely cut out sweets, cold turkey that January – after the holidays. I ate smaller meals comprised mostly of green leafy vegetables, fish, and fruit – meat hadn't part of my diet for over 20 years, so that wasn't a concern. I drank 2 eight-ounce glasses of lemon water daily. Finally, I started interval training 5 times a week. The result at my next medical check-in 3 months later was that I had lost 40 pounds going from 212 pounds to 172 pounds – my wife thought I lost too much weight. However, most important, my blood pressure was 115 over 70 and my blood sugar level was in the perfect range. I continue to live my new lifestyle to this very day, enjoying sweets on occasion. I thank the Creator for giving me the wisdom, understanding, and will power to change my life. This book is part of my testimony.

The fountain of youth has been the quest of many people over the span of time. Although the secret to restore immediate youth hasn't been discovered, we have the power to slow aging and stay healthy. I believe it's possible for human beings to live healthy productive lives well into the 110's or 120's. Some may question the notion that a person can live a quality life well into the 100's, especially, if they are dealing with health challenges, chronic fatigue or haven't taken care of themselves for years. My response is that it's never too late to get started. Most illness, including major causes of death and suffering, such as heart disease, cancer, respiratory disease, stroke, Alzheimer's, and diabetes can be avoided by eating a well-balanced healthy diet and being active daily. By eating well and exercising daily you may be able to slow the aging process and possibly reverse the effects of aging.

What would you pay to feel and appear younger, have more energy, be disease free and have an overall better quality of life? I'm sure you agree, it's priceless. I submit that all I describe in this book is possible for you and the people you love, if you live the way the Creator intended. Let's explore the process together to become a more healthy and vital you, poised to live a longer, better-quality life – you deserve it.

CHAPTER 1:
AVOID THE CAUSES OF ILLNESS

In the past, life was much simpler. Remember the days when there was a family garden in the back yard. The garden was planted in spring, managed throughout summer – with some fresh fruit and vegetables gathered in the warm months, but the bounty harvested in the fall. Most food was eaten, but some was jarred or canned for the winter months. Nice, fresh, and healthy food -- those were the days. People lived a more healthy and natural lifestyle.

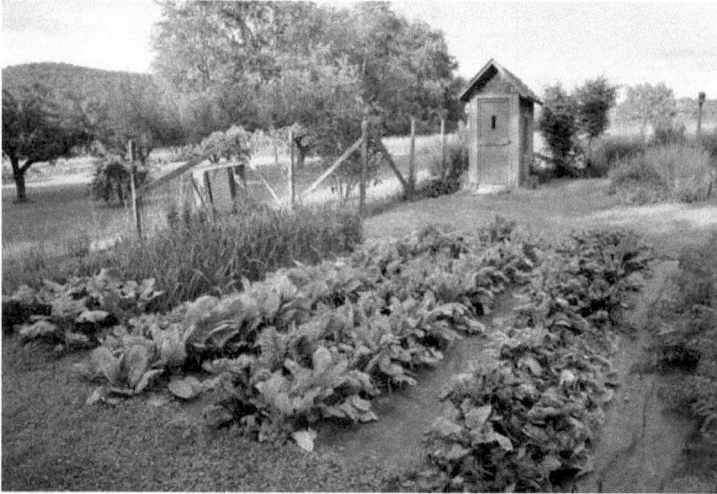

Fast forward, advancements in food processing have given us more food choices than ever before that are easily available, fast, and convenient. You can heat up a TV dinner, order at the fast food drive through window or get a meal at a fast-casual restaurant. But, unfortunately, many of these foods we eat are processed. Processed foods contribute to the acidic content in your body, causing your body to change to an unhealthy acidic state. A highly acidic diet causes your cells and organs to function abnormally, causing inflammation, and illness in the body. Most non-vegetarian foods are highly acidic in nature. Sweets, salty foods, red meats, chicken, egg yolks, white rice, and white bread all contribute to the acidic content in the body that has been attributed to the rampant growth of heart disease, diabetes, cancer, high blood pressure, kidney disease and even Alzheimer's disease.

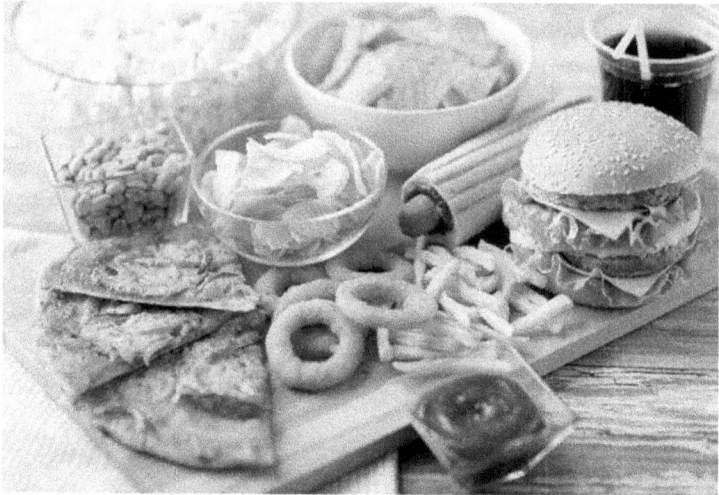

Highly acidic foods lead to premature aging of cells in the body including hair loss, wrinkling of the skin, poor skin condition and tooth decay. Further, highly acidic foods lead to sickness, disease, fatigue, and a general feeling of persistent tiredness. First things first – to begin to change your body's acidic state, you first need to detoxify.

How to Detoxify

The creator designed the human body to remarkably heal itself when it is in the right state and the proper conditions exist. When you take medicine, shower with tap water, consume candy, eat sugary baked goods, eat red meat, eat fried foods, inhale car exhaust, drink alcohol, smoke cigarettes, or use cleaning products without gloves, you are increasing your body's toxicity level. In addition to external toxins, our bodies create internal toxins from breathing and eating. If toxins are not filtered via the liver and kidneys, routed through the lymphatic system for elimination through urination, bowel movements, sweat through the skin, or mucus via the mouth; they wound up circulating in the bloodstream, stored in fat cells, organs, and connective tissue of organs. Over time, our body's turn into toxic repositories that are open to all manner of diseases.

What are the next steps to detoxify? Just as you need to change the oil in your car every 3,000 miles to avoid slug build-up in the engine, you need to detoxify your body every three (3) months. Moreover, you should change your life style and eating habits, so that you're detoxifying daily. Most toxins can be eliminated by eating detoxifying foods that are nutritious and fibrous such as green leafy vegetables, fresh fruit, beans, and whole grains that are cooked in the least amount of time possible to retain the most nutrients. Certain vegetables contain key nutrients to aid the liver in detoxifying blood in the body, but break down if cooked too long. Some of the best detoxifying vegetables and fruit include garlic, onions, broccoli, cabbage, cauliflower, green tea, and lemons.

Another great method to detoxify the body is through fasting, which I cover in detail later in the book. How does fasting work? Fasting is the process of not eating any solid foods, while drinking filtered water, spring water or certain juices for a set duration of time to allow the body the opportunity to cleanse itself. Consequently, this triggers the body's healing process.

Other methods to detoxify include colonics. First let's look at the root causes for toxins in the colon. When the colon accumulates undigested foods, toxins begin to form in the intestinal wall laying the foundation for disease. Challenges such as flatulence, belching, constipation, indigestion, food cravings, headaches, fatigue, allergies, yeast, and irritable bowel syndrome (IBS) are some of the symptoms of toxic build-up. These conditions signal an imbalance in the colon.

What are colonics? Colon irrigation, also known as colon hydrotherapy, is an effective process that flushes the large intestine with warm filtered water, sometimes mixed with herbs, to loosen and remove accumulated waste on the colon walls. Colonics clean the colon using multiple infusions and usually lasts for an hour. After a colonic, it's important to restore friendly bacteria by eating Greek yogurt or other colon healthy foods.

Another popular and famous detox program is called the Master Cleanse. This program requires that you only drink a combination of lemon juice, maple syrup, cayenne pepper and water for a short period of time averaging about 10 days; however, I recommend 2 to 3 days to get started. This formula is claimed to provide all the required nutrition the body needs to operate. Another detox method is a warm Epson salt bath or foot soak to extract toxins from your body.

Another key part of detoxification is getting regular daily exercise. Do whatever you want – walking, running, biking, housework -- just stay active. I know you've heard a million times that exercise is good for you. Why? Let's explore the reason exercise is good for you. According to the Mayo Clinic, the health

benefits of regular exercise and physical activity
cannot be ignored. Regardless of age, gender or
ability, everyone can benefit from regular
exercise. I list the benefits for you below:

- *Controls weight*: Exercise can help
  prevent excess weight gain or help
  maintain weight loss. When you engage in
  physical activity, you burn calories.

- *Combats health conditions and diseases*:
  exercise boosts high-density lipoprotein
  (HDL), or "good," cholesterol and
  decreases unhealthy triglycerides.
  Exercise keeps your blood flowing
  smoothly, which decreases your risk of

cardiovascular diseases. Regular exercise helps prevent or manage a wide range of health problems and concerns, including stroke, metabolic syndrome, Type 2 diabetes, depression, arthritis, and falls.

- *Exercise improves mood:* Physical activity stimulates various brain chemicals that make you feel happier and more relaxed.

- *Exercise boosts energy:* Regular physical activity improves muscle strength and increases your endurance. Exercise increases delivery of oxygen and nutrients to your cells and helps your cardiovascular system work better. When your heart and lung health improve, you have more energy to tackle daily activities.

- *Promotes better sleep:* Regular physical activity can help you fall asleep faster and deepen your sleep.

- *Increases your sex drive:* Regular physical activity can improve energy levels and physical appearance, which may boost your sex life. Regular physical activity may enhance arousal for women, and men who exercise regularly are less likely to have problems with erectile dysfunction than men who don't exercise.

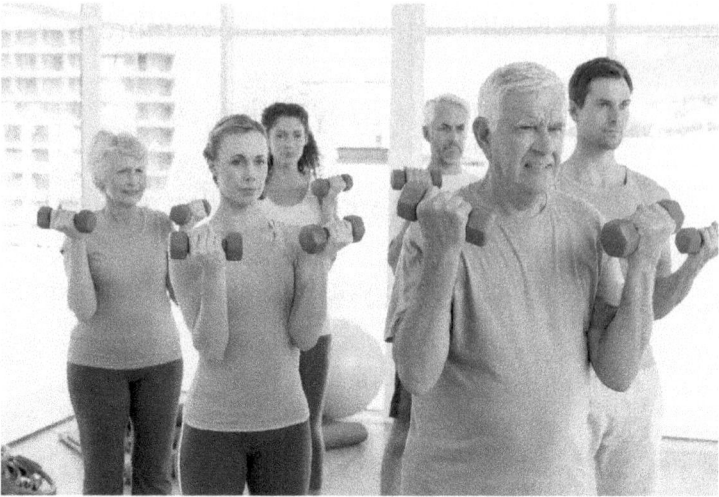

When you exercise it causes your heart to beat faster; increases circulation which opens your arteries and veins for improved blood flow, so more blood and nutrients flow to your cells and brain. It also enhances lymphatic system performance, which is the body's waste drainage system, to work better assisting in detoxification of the body.

Additional benefits of exercise include improving the body's immune system by increasing the white blood cell performance and ridding toxins from the body through sweat.

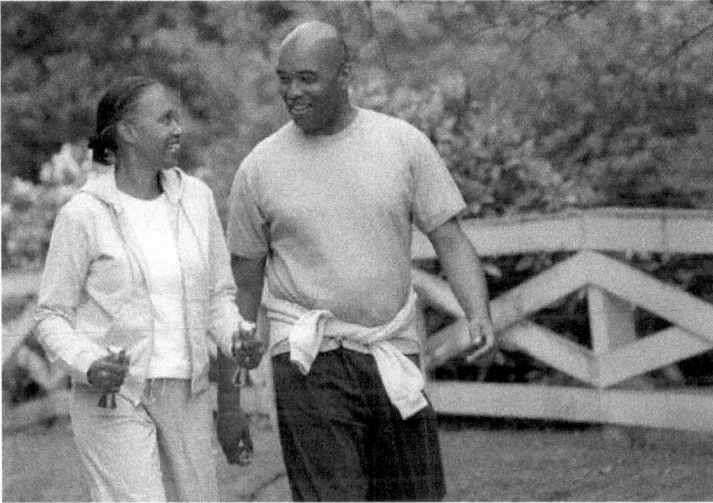

Try to get at least 30 minutes of moderate-intensity exercise, or 30 minutes of interval exercise, three (3) times per week.

CHAPTER 2:
ANCIENT HEALING AND
WEIGHT LOSS METHOD

It is widely accepted that disease may be the result of the build-up of toxins in our bodies, resulting in inflammation. Fortunately, the answer to heal disease has been re-discovered. It is an ancient method that has been practiced for thousands of years, but was lost with modern medicine and the current fast pace of life. In addition to eliminating disease in the body, some added benefits to this method is weight loss, lower blood pressure, slower aging, more energy, faster healing, better sleep, sharper thinking, clearer skin, healthier hair, fresher breath, stronger finger nails, clearer eyes, etc. This ancient method has also been referenced in the Bible:

"But when you fast, put oil on your head and wash your face, so that it will not be obvious to others that you are fasting, but only to your Father, who is unseen; and your Father, who sees what is done in secret, will reward you".

Matthew 6:17-18

Yes, the ancient healing and weight loss method is Fasting. What is Fasting?

Fasting gives the body a chance to cleanse itself and begin healing. For most people, a short fast of 3 to 5 days is recommended to get started. However, interesting things start to happen during a 30 day fast. During the first 2 to 3 days, the body eliminates toxins through urination and bowel movements, and the blood begins the cleansing process. Since enzymes and helper cells are not needed by the stomach and colon, their attention turns to destroying diseased cells, pathogens in the blood and purging toxins from the body. From days 5 to 10, the immune system begins to heal and rebuild itself, because the body is not in a constant battle with pathogens. In the period from days 11 to 30, diseases begin to reverse, and the body develops a healthier balanced state. At day 30, according to Herbert Shelton, a known practitioner of water fasting who supervised 35,000 fasts between 1925 to 1970, serious illness and disease begin to disappear. In addition, it has been reported that there is a reversal of the signs of aging, reduced high cholesterol, high blood pressure, headaches, digestive problems, obesity, arthritis, heart disease, cysts, fibroids, and benign tumors.

Mini Fast

The Mini Fast entails eating only 2 meals within an 8-hour period, say between 10am and

6pm. During this fast, your body receives the nourishment in requires, your blood sugar is balanced, and you maintain lower hunger levels without feeling deprived of food. The Mini Fast also allows you to kickstart weight loss by eating less calories per day.

Once a fast is complete, you must govern yourself by eating healthy foods, cutting out processed foods, sugar, sweet drinks, reducing stress, stop excess alcohol consumption, eliminate smoking, as well as, drinking 6 to 8 glasses of water daily.

Water fasting for example, has been used to detoxify the body for thousands of years. It has been reported to reverse many signs of aging, reduce bad cholesterol levels, reduce high blood pressure, eliminate cysts, and stomach problems, lower weight, reduce heart disease risk and headaches – and many other conditions.

Today, you should be careful when going on a water only Fast due to the high pollution levels in our tap water. If you try the water only Fast, you should use only bottled spring or fortified mineral water for short periods of time – 2 to 3 days, then build up over time. <u>Very important</u>, if you have health conditions, let your doctor know that you intend to Fast in advance. Another Fast is the Juice Fast.

The Juice Fast

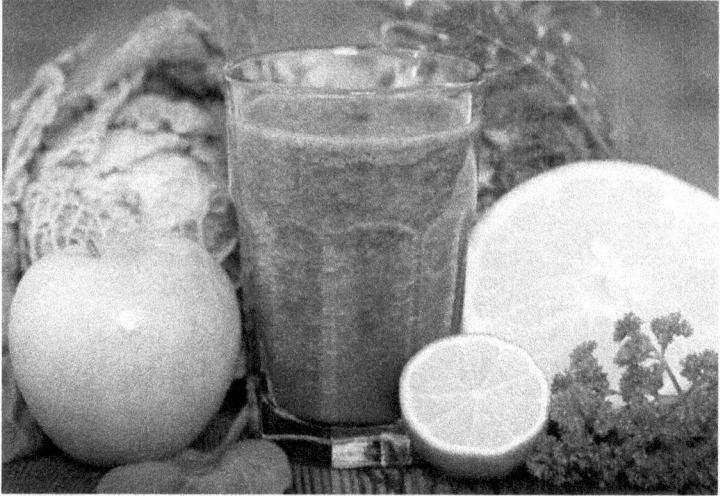

Juice Fasting produces effective cleansing results, with health benefits comparable to water-only Fasts. Juice has an added benefit of providing enzymes for detoxification that our stressed liver needs in extra amounts. During a juice fast, no solid food is eaten, use a combination of apple, carrot, grape, beet, celery, or cabbage. Don't use orange or tomatoes, because they are too acidic. Note the following below:

- A 24-hour juice Fast will eliminate toxins.

- A 3-day juice Fast will start to cleanse the blood and help the body eliminate toxins.

- A 5-day juice fast will cleanse the blood, eliminate toxins, burn fat, and begin healing diseases – work up to this level slowly.

Eat Detoxifying Foods for Spring Cleaning

Give your body a spring cleaning by eating foods that sweep the intestine clean. This means eating foods that are high in fiber such as fresh fruit and vegetables, whole grains, and beans (e.g., black and kidney). Try to eat these foods raw, if possible, or steamed for just a few minutes. If possible, cease eating all meat while detoxifying to make your body more alkaline.

Eat fruit such as apples, apricots, melons, berries, and other fruit, which are all high alkaline foods and have fiber. If you have digestive problems, eat lightly cooked fruit, which is gentler on the stomach.

In addition, drink lemon water to cleanse your system. Although lemon is acidic on its own, when digested it has an alkalizing effect on the body. It simple - just squeeze half of a fresh lemon into a glass of water and drink twice daily.

HEALTH BENEFITS OF DRINKING LEMON WATER

Lemon is a natural energizer; it hydrates & oxygenates the body so it feels revitalized & refreshed!

Boosts your immune system
Balance pH
Flush out unwanted materials
Decrease wrinkles & blemishes
Relieve tooth pain
Relieves respiratory problems
Cures Throat Infections
Excellent for Weight Loss
Reduces Fever
Blood purifier

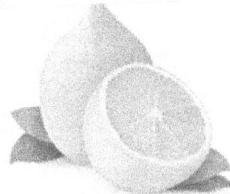

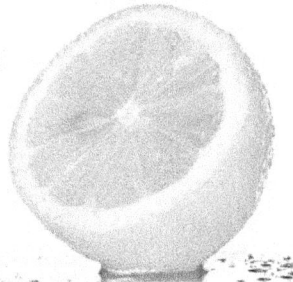

Eat more alkalizing greens, such as kale, turnips, mustard greens, endive, and collard greens, which all increase alkalinity. Eat at least two cups of greens per day.

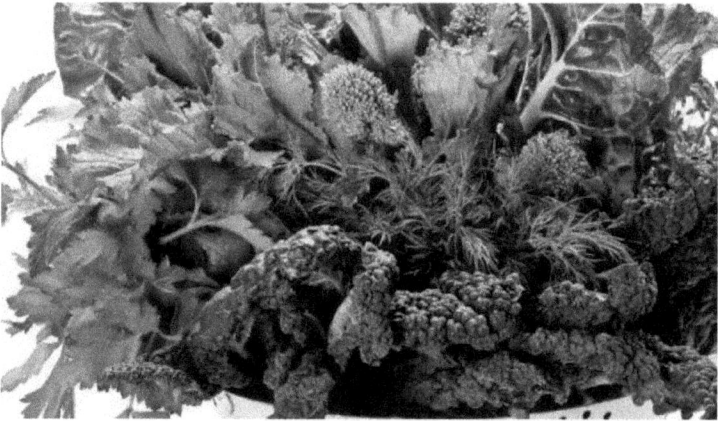

Seaweed also makes the body more alkaline, and should be eaten often. Add oats, brown rice, quinoa, yams, sweet potatoes, and lentils to your diet as well.

Exercise to Detox

Add a regular exercise program to your routine that includes walking, jogging, light weight lifting or exercise classes for thirty minutes, three times a week. Always consult your physician before starting new programs.

In short, eat clean and live well. Try to eat organic foods that are free of pesticides or genetic changes, avoid polluted areas, live where the air is cleaner. Ensure you change the air filters every 3 month to improve the air quality in your home. Detoxify your body, eat alkaline foods, and regain your health the natural way.

CHAPTER 3:
FOOD IS YOUR MEDICINE,
MEDICINE IS YOUR FOOD

"Let food be thy medicine and
medicine be thy food."
Hippocrates, "The father of medicine"

Your Food is Your Medicine

Long before modern medicine, Hippocrates who lived from 466 to 377 BC and considered the founding father of medicine, believed that illness was a natural event that forced people to discover the imbalances in their health. He strongly believed in good food and related the development of any ailment to poor nutrition and bad lifestyle habits. He stressed, "Let food be your medicine and medicine be your food." Also, according to biblical scripture in Genesis 2:7, "the Lord formed man from the dust of the ground and breathed into his nostrils the breath of life, and man became a living being." Therefore, it is reasonable to assume that the Creator would ensure that the food eaten by man from the earth would contain everything required to sustain and keep him healthy.

Research that reinforces the power of food to treat or reverse disease is beginning to grow. In addition, doctors are looking at the cumulative data on diet and a clear picture is emerging - salt,

39

sugar, fat, and processed foods in the American diet contribute to the nation's very high rate of obesity, cancer, diabetes, and heart disease. Per the World Health Organization, 80 percent of deaths from heart disease and stroke are caused by high blood pressure, tobacco use, elevated cholesterol and low consumption of fruit and vegetables.

With that said, to establish a healthy and balanced life, you must return to the way the Creator intended by eating healthy and exercising your body daily. Let's explore the foods that are your medicine and components of a healthy diet.

As noted earlier, the western diet, largely comprised of processed food, provides little nutritional value, and I believe, leads to the development of a lot of the diseases today. How can you change your diet to become more healthy and balanced? The solution to a more balanced diet is to eat clean, which includes eating unprocessed foods along with some acidic foods to get the pH level in the body to neutral.

The foundation of a healthy diet is a high nutrient, low calorie diet comprised primarily of fresh vegetables, fruits, herbs that are locally organically grown, if possible. The key ingredients in vegetables, fruits, and herbs that the human body loves are called phytochemicals, which are defined as plant based. It is essential to eat a lot of vegetables, such as kale, collard greens, broccoli, spinach, lettuce, cauliflower, radish, carrots, peas, eggplant, etc. Consume at least two cups of alkalizing greens per day. You could add oats, wild rice, quinoa, yams, sweet potatoes, and lentils to your diet, as well.

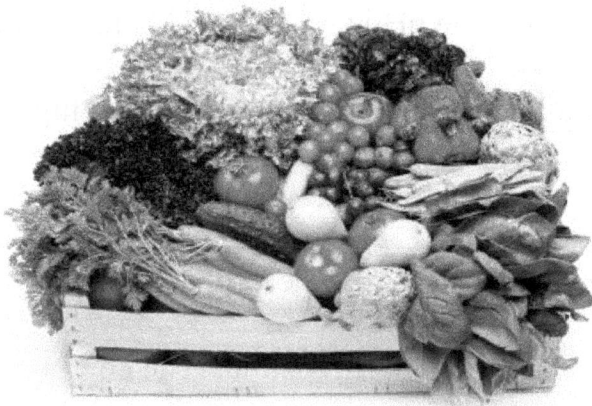

Also eat plenty of fruit such as apples, blueberries, pears, peaches, oranges, watermelon, pineapple, plums, kiwi, etc. A simple solution for those who love to eat meats is to combine them with vegetables to get a balance. For example, eat chicken with broccoli and sweet potato to get a balance. In general, it may be noted that-

- About 75 % of total food intake should be alkaline in nature. This is most essential for proper digestion and good health.
- Alkaline foods lead to a more active brain and sharper thinking.

43

- Alkaline foods lead to an active body, which is less prone to headaches, colds, and illnesses.

- A highly alkaline diet slows down the process of aging, increases energy and is highly recommended for young looking skin and improved vision.

How to Make the Body More Alkaline

Reduce the amount of sugar and meat consumed in your diet. Sugar and meat is acid-forming foods and raises the acidity level of the body. If possible, cease eating all sugar and meat, while changing your diet to make your body more alkaline quicker.

Try to make vegetables and fruits two-thirds of your daily diet. As noted, green leafy vegetables, berries and other fruit are all high alkaline foods. Fresh fruit juice is equally important and may be consumed. However, be careful not to drink too much fruit juice due to the high sugar content. If you have digestive problems, concentrate on eating cooked vegetables and fruit, which is gentler on the stomach, but will still make your body alkaline. Take vitamin and mineral supplements that increases alkalinity, such as Vitamin C and magnesium to raise the alkalinity in the body.

When taking these supplements, follow the

recommended dosage information.

The Healing Power of Green Tea

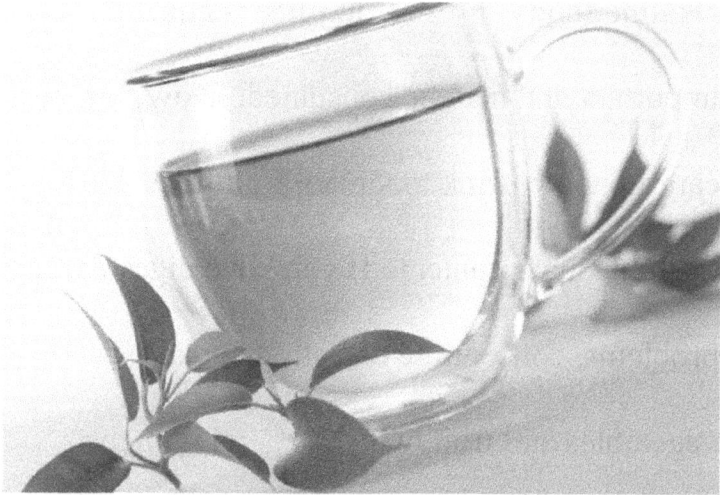

I was first introduced to green tea in the early

1990's in Washington D.C. by Ms. Holbrook,

who I lovingly called my grandmother. She

worked at the US National Arboretum and had a

deep knowledge of plants and herbs. Mother

46

Holbrook explained that green tea had a lot of health benefits to help me stay healthy and that it would be a good idea to make green tea part of my daily diet. I fully embraced that wisdom and my love with green tea began. Mother Holbrook was 76 at the time and lived for another 22 healthy years. I didn't fully know the great healing power of green tea until I started digging deeper into its history and the many health benefits it offered. Fast forward, I've been drinking 1 to 2 cups of green tea, without sweeteners, daily for the past 26 years, and can personally attest to the health benefits green tea offers. Let me explain further.

The earliest recorded history of green tea use dates back 4,000 years in China. The Chinese believed that green tea would ward off disease, increase vitality, and enhance health. Growing U.S. scientific research is confirming that herbs and specifically green tea contain many health promoting and healing compounds for sustained health. Researchers call these compounds phytonutrients, ("phyto", the Greek word for plant, and "nutrient", nourishment essential for growth and maintenance of life), which are naturally occurring compounds found in plants. Plants use these compounds for protection and survival from parasites, bacteria, free radicals, viruses, insects and injures. Therefore, it is reasonable to assume that the Creator in his infinite wisdom intended that those benefits and protections would transfer to humans when we consumed plants, to include green tea.

Some of the health benefits purported from drinking 3 cups of green tea a day include quicker healing, improved blood flow, disease prevention, heart health, detoxification, boosting immunity, better digestion, healthy teeth, and gums, enhanced mental clarity, younger looking skin, sharper eyesight, fatigue elimination, lower blood sugar and a better state of being.

What are the secret ingredients in green tea?

I'm glad you asked. Well, they are polyphenols, caffeine, nutrients, and aromatic oils – each play a vital role in the health benefits and taste of green tea. The first compound are polyphenols, which occur naturally in tea and are responsible for tea's pungent favor and powerful antioxidant property. Green tea's color is due to chlorophyll and polyphenols. The antioxidants are the components that are responsible for disease prevention and treatment. The second component, caffeine, is a stimulant found in small amounts in green tea. The third component in green tea are nutrients that contain vitamins and minerals found in small amounts.

The final component are aromatic oils, which contribute to the flavor and aroma of tea.

How much green tea should you drink daily? In order to get the maximum benefits, you should drink 2 to 4 cups (8 fluid ounces or 237 milligrams) of green tea daily.

One study in Japan followed 3,380 Japanese women for nine years, who drank green tea 6 times a day. The findings where remarkable. These women were at least 50 years old and were members of a Japanese tea ceremony. They tracked the mortality rate of these women from 1980 through 1988 and found that a smaller percentage of women in this group got sick or died, compared to other women throughout Japan in the same age group, suggesting that the protective components of green tea reduced the occurrence of disease or fatal conditions. Green tea's role in health are many. Let's review:

Condition	Green Tea benefits
Diabetes	Promotes normal blood sugar and insulin regulation
Heart Disease	Lowers bad LDL cholesterol and blood pressure, as well as, prevents platelet sticking
Weak Immune System	Boosts immune and anti-microbial properties
Toxin Buildup	Aids the liver and kidney to function better to remove toxins from the body
Poor Mental Function	Helps to promote cognitive functions to include

	improved memory and sharpness
Poor Circulation	Helps to improve blood circulation and lowers risk of hardening of the arteries
Cancer	May reduce the risk developing various cancers to include breast, skin, and colon cancers

Let me be clear that green tea is not a cure all, rather, what I'm suggesting that a combination of drinking green tea 3-times daily, eating a well-balanced diet that includes plenty of green vegetables and exercising by walking, running, swimming, biking, and lifting light weights at least 3-times a week, will lead to a long healthier and diseased free life.

CHAPTER 4:

THE DIET THAT MAY CUT YOUR RISK
OF DEVELOPING ALZHEIMER'S

Wouldn't it be great if the way we ate could stay off aging diseases like Alzheimer's? Well, I have great news for you, it's true – the better you eat, the less likely you are to develop debilitating diseases like Alzheimer's. Let's explore what it takes.

There has been talk for years about how eating green leafy veggies, berries and nuts can help keep you healthy and your mind alert. But now there's medical science to back it up and living proof as well. These foods are known as brain healthy foods.

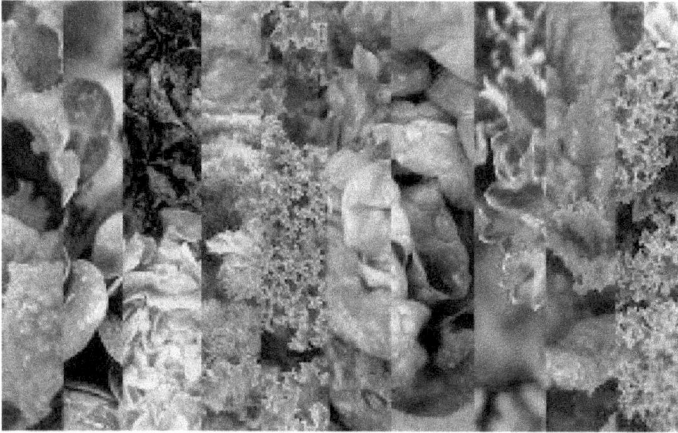

Experts say there is increased awareness that lifestyle factors, not just genetics, play a prominent role in the development of Alzheimer's. An estimated 5.1 million people in the U.S. have Alzheimer's, a number expected to grow to 7.1 million by 2025, according to the Alzheimer's Association.

As I noted in the last chapter, your food is your medicine and your medicine is your food. It is my firm belief that nutrition can improve brain health and stave off the cognitive decline and memory impairment that comes with Alzheimer's disease and other forms of dementia. According to WebMD, folic acid found in leafy green vegetables, citrus fruits, and beans may be effective to prevent memory loss, Alzheimer's disease, age-related hearing loss, preventing the eye disease Age-related Macular Degeneration (AMD), reducing signs of aging, weak bones (osteoporosis). So, what is this diet?

The diet is a variation of the Mediterranean diet, which includes elements of the following foods:

- Green leafy veggies: It is well known by doctors that deficiencies of certain B vitamins and folate found in dark leafy greens has been associated with declining mental sharpness. Low levels of these vitamins and folate impairs the brain function and can significantly increase a person's risk of developing Alzheimer's disease as well as heart disease. These foods below have many beneficial effects:

- o Kale, Collard greens, Turnip greens, Swiss chard, Spinach, Mustard greens, Broccoli, Green leaf lettuce, Romaine lettuce, and Cabbage

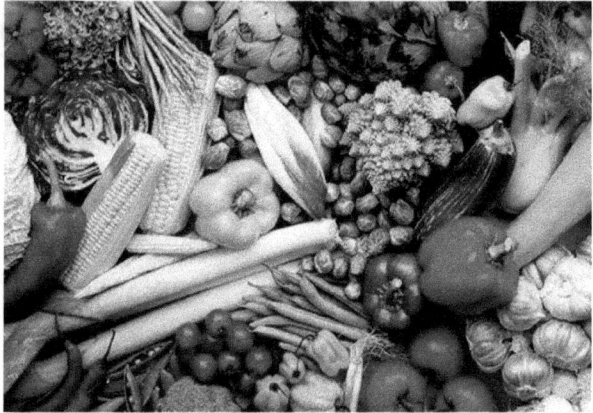

- Fruit:
  - o Apples, pears, oranges, blueberries, watermelon, peaches, kiwi, papaya, cantaloupe, strawberries, bananas, and pineapple

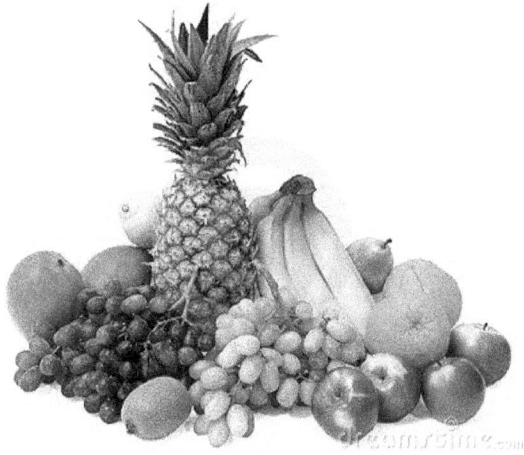

- Nuts:

  o Almonds, Walnuts, Hazelnuts.

    Cashews, Pistachios, Peanuts,

    Pecans

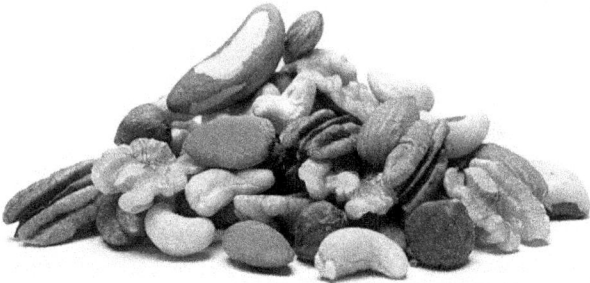

- Berries:

  - Blueberries, Goji Berries, Acai Berries, Strawberries. Blackberries, Cherries

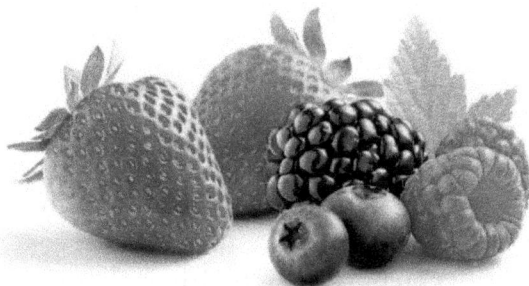

- Beans: beans are good for your heart, have cholesterol-clobbering fiber, and contain plenty of potassium.

- o Green, red kidney, cannellini, black, navy, garbanzo, lima, pea, lentil, pigeon pea, peanut, pinto

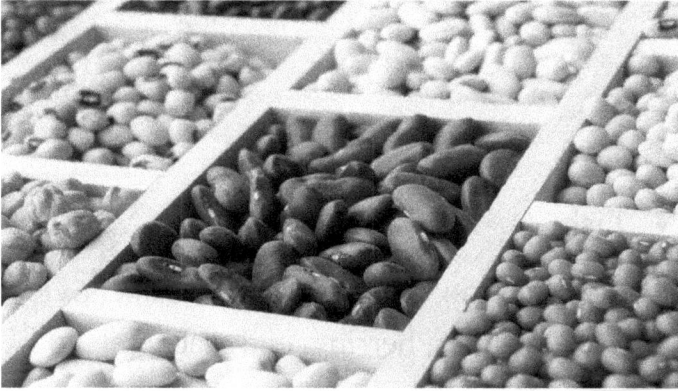

- Whole Grains
  - o Barley, Buckwheat, Corn, Oats, Quinoa, Brown rice, Wheat, Wild rice

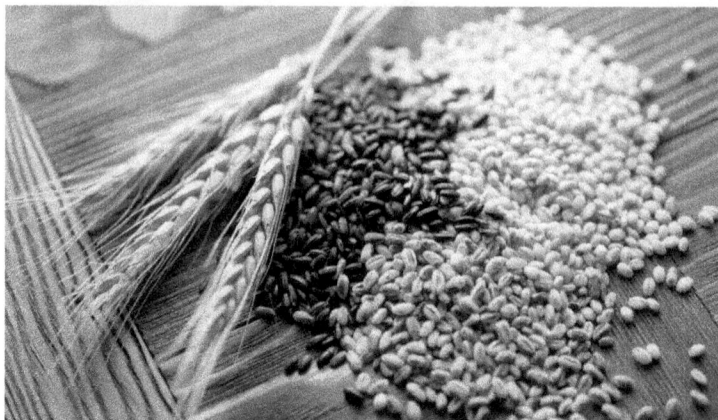

- Fish

  - Salmon, small fish such as anchovies, sardines, herring, and mackerel

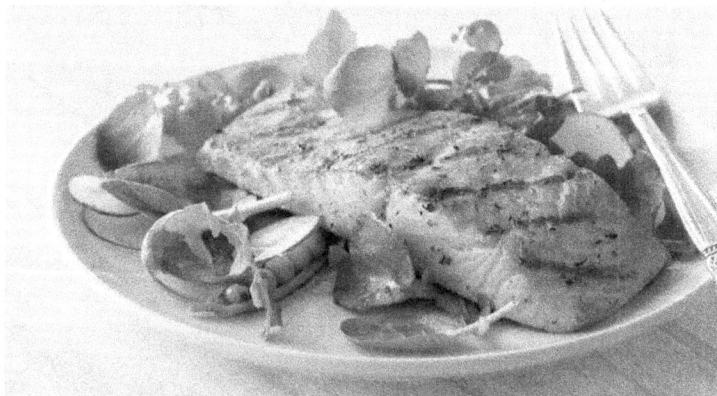

- Olive Oil – Extra virgin

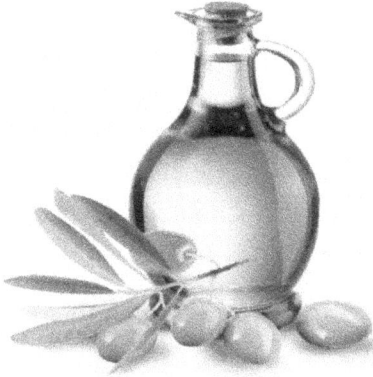

- Wine: One (1) glass of red wine daily

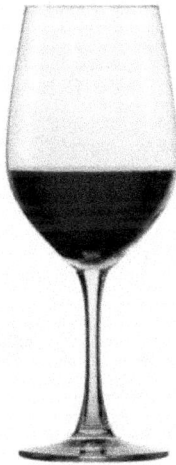

The Anti-Alzheimer's diet includes eating at least two servings of plant-based foods, such as leafy green vegetables and fruits, whole grains, legumes and nuts every day - along with a glass of red wine and 6 to 8 glasses of water daily.

The diet also involves snacking most days on nuts or fruit, and eating beans every other day or so, berries at least twice a week and fish (for example salmon or sardines) at least twice a week. I can't emphasize enough that people should eat green leafy vegetables at least twice a day. The body efficiently processes green vegetables and aids in cellular restoration, especially in the intestinal track. In addition, greens are the true Brain food by helping the brain restore cells, as well as, maintain and enhance brain function.

In India and other countries that cook with curry, people have a lower occurrence of Alzheimer's than in Western countries. Curry powder could be the reason for the lower risk. The key ingredient in curry powder is turmeric, which contains curcumin (the component that gives curry its yellowish color). Research conducted on lab animals given curcumin found that they have improved memory in tests. Curcumin is a powerful antioxidant, anti-inflammatory, and anti-amyloid compound (note: amyloid compound is composed of amino acids that are critically involved in Alzheimer's disease and is the main component of the amyloid plaque found in the brains of Alzheimer patients). To be effective, include two tablespoons of curry in soups or your favorite bean dishes.

Another remarkable herb that has been used for centuries to improve memory and mental sharpness is Sage. Medical research is underway and Sage appears to be effective in protecting acetylcholine, which is an organic chemical that functions in the brain as a neurotransmitter to send signals to other brain cells. Some human trials found that Sage or its oil improved memory and cognitive function. Sage may also have anti-inflammatory benefits that help slow the progression of Alzheimer's. You can add sage to your food or add two teaspoons of dried sage to boiling water for a healthy cup of sage tea.

The key to maintaining good brain health is to eat healthy plant based foods, while eliminating sugar, excess salt, fat, processed foods, and toxins from the body. I believe green leafy vegetables protect the body by preventing the buildup of fatty deposits in the brain and liver, which can lead to brain cell destruction and plaque buildup.

Also, green leafy vegetables promote daily bowel movements to eliminate toxins and fat from the body. One should have at least 2 bowel movements daily. Key note, one way to tell your body is eliminating fat is when you see bowel movement floating.

Don't forget to drink at least 6 to 8 glasses of water daily. Water keeps everything moving throughout your body. It helps move toxins through the lymphatic system, which you can think of as the body's cesspool. Through the process of digestion, the kidneys and liver filter the blood coming from the digestive tract to eliminate toxins, and the colon transforms food into a fuel source for cells or stored in fat cells for later use.

A bonus from eating plenty of vegetables is that it not only reduces the risk of developing Alzheimer's, but reduces stroke and heart disease risk, as well. Certain foods are considered unhealthy and may in fact contribute to developing Alzheimer's disease. Baby Boomers and everyone else as well, should make it a point to avoid eating the following foods on a daily basis:

- Poultry
- Red Meats
- Butter and margarine

69

- Cheese

- Pastries, cakes, candy, and sweets

- Fried foods

- Fast food

- Processed foods

I can't emphasize enough that you must limit eating the designated unhealthy foods, especially white sugar, candy, butter, cheese, fried foods, and fast food to avoid developing the devastating effects of Alzheimer's.

CHAPTER 5:
NATURAL METHODS TO
LOWER BLOOD PRESSURE

High blood pressure can lead to dangerous consequences like heart attacks, strokes, and kidney failure. It is estimated that High blood pressure, also called hypertension, affects about 1 in 4 adults, or 75 million Americans, and 30% of African Americans under the age of 50 have high blood pressure in the United States.

Here are a few natural remedies that can be used to control and reduce it:

Garlic is thought to be one of the most

effective remedies against high blood pressure.

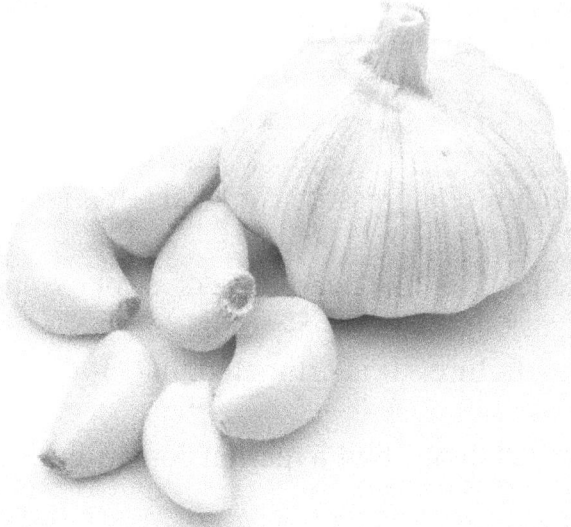

Clinical research has proven that fresh garlic and garlic supplements have the ability of destroying plaque, preventing blood clots, and lowering bad cholesterol levels. According to a clinical study conducted by the National Institutes of Health in 2014, it was found that when high blood pressure patients were given a single garlic clove per day for twelve weeks, it resulted in a significant reduction of their cholesterol levels, as well as, a lower diastolic blood pressure (lower number). However, garlic supplements ought to be taken under medical supervision, since it acts in a similar manner as aspirin by thinning the blood or reducing the bloods ability to clot.

Please note, garlic could also interfere with supplements like vitamin E and Gingko, as well as, prescription drugs, such as blood thinning medications Pentoxifylline (Trental), and Warfarin (Coumadin).

What about fish oil? Recent research

supports the efficacy of fish oil having a beneficial effect on high blood pressure. It has been shown when individuals with hypertension took fish oil supplements equivalent to 5-15 grams per day, it resulted in a significant lowering of blood pressure. According to another research study by the National Institutes of Health, having a low dosage of fish oil daily was proven to be helpful for reducing blood pressure in patients with mild hypertension.

Folic acid is a B vitamin, which is essential for the formation of red blood cells. Folate occurs naturally in many foods, but especially green leafy vegetables, beans, and citrus fruits. It can be used for preventing stroke associated with high blood pressure, and treating low blood levels of folate (folate deficiency), as well as its complications, including "tired blood" (anemia) and the inability of the gastrointestinal tract to absorb nutrients properly. Folic acid is also used for other conditions commonly associated with ulcerative colitis, liver disease, alcoholism, and kidney dialysis. According to WebMD, Folic acid is used for jumpy legs (restless leg syndrome), sleep problems, depression, nerve pain, muscle pain, a skin disease called vitiligo, and an inherited disease called Fragile-X syndrome. Foods that are naturally high in folate include spinach, broccoli, lettuce, okra, asparagus, bananas, melons, lemons, beans, yeast, mushrooms, orange juice, and tomato juice. In a study conducted on cigarette smokers, who were given a supplement of folic acid for four weeks, it significantly reduced their blood pressure.

These days, aromatherapy is increasingly being used as a natural remedy for high blood pressure. Blue chamomile could be inhaled directly to counter stress. Massaged on the collarbone each night with a combination of sunflower oil, blue chamomile oil and lavender oil may help relieve tension.

Celery oil and celery help to dilate muscles, which helps in regulating blood pressure.

A large worldwide study revealed when potassium is balanced in relation to sodium, blood pressure was lower. Potassium allows the body to get rid of extra fluid, so that the heart does not have to pump as hard, thereby allowing blood pressure to stay low. It is also important for regulating the heart-beat. Good sources of potassium include most fruits and vegetables, especially apricots, oranges, bananas, sweet potatoes, and tomatoes. It's important to note that too much potassium can be detrimental by causing changes in your heart rhythm.

Magnesium is another important mineral for keeping blood pressure under control. Good sources of magnesium include dark green vegetables, nuts, seeds, and legumes.

Calcium has many interesting health benefits beyond strengthening bones. People who include more calcium in their foods tend to have lower blood pressure, weigh less, less body fat, and have a lower risk for developing type 2 diabetes. There are many vegetables that are good sources of calcium such as almond milk, that is formulated to be good sources of calcium. Taking a calcium supplement and lowering the intake of salt are also beneficial.

Medical science has found that hypertension can also be caused by free radicals, and that a daily dosage of vitamin C can lower blood pressure significantly in those who are afflicted with hypertension. Vitamin C is found naturally in red peppers, oranges, kale, broccoli, brussel sprouts, strawberries, guava, and kiwi.

Exercise

High blood pressure can also be controlled by making lifestyle changes. Enhance the benefits of healthy eating by adding a regular exercise program at least 30 minutes a day, 3 times a week that may include walking, jogging, light weight lifting or exercise classes. Always consult your physician before starting any new programs to ensure you can safely exercise. Reduce your blood pressure the natural way and enjoy a healthier you.

CHAPTER 6:
NATURE'S HEALERS:
GARLIC AND ONIONS

Garlic and onions have a very long history as powerful healing foods that are effective against all types of ailments and diseases. Every health promoting diet should include liberal amounts of garlic and onions either raw or cooked lightly. You can include them in salads, seafood, vegetables, stews, soups, and spreads to infuse these foods with their potent and delicious flavor.

ReGenesis: Living the Way the Creator Intended

The Power of Garlic

Garlic has been a widely-used ailment remedy for over 3000 years. It has been used to treat colds, asthma, high cholesterol, high blood pressure, diabetes, and flu. Garlic is an immune system boosting food containing twelve or more antioxidants, which include two of the most important ones, zinc and selenium.

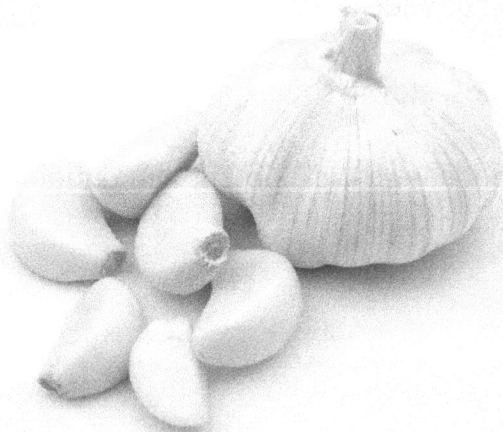

82

Garlic also has anticancer properties that stimulate the body's production of natural disease killer cells, which may destroy the cancer cells and pathogens that attack healthy cells in your body.

Not only does garlic taste good, it has antibacterial, antiviral, anti-fungal and anti-inflammatory properties, as well. People who have suffered from an infection of the digestive system, who ate one to four cloves of raw garlic daily, improved their digestive track and rid their intestines of pathogens, while leaving the good bacteria unharmed. Also, studies have shown that eating garlic may cut the risk of colorectal and stomach cancer by up to half.

Thank the Creator for Onions

Onions help protect the heart by lowering blood pressure and preventing blood clots, as well as, boosting the immune system. They also may have powerful anticancer properties that block cancer cell production. Onions are also effective against Salmonella and E.coli.

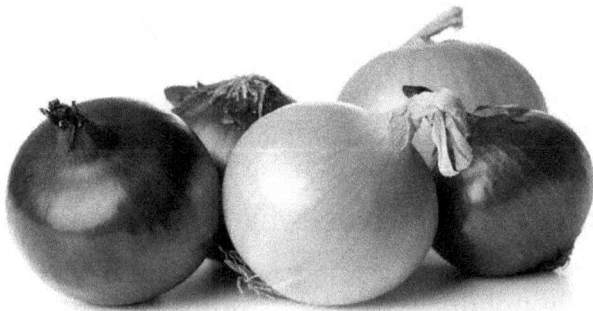

Onions, however, are not as potent as Garlic at fighting these bugs, because it has a lower level of sulfur compounds that is one quarter the level of Garlic.

How to use Garlic and Onions Everyday

Garlic and onions are inexpensive and offer an easy way to add flavor to your food, so use them liberally. There are many kinds of onions ranging from green onions, scallions, leeks, red onions, white onions, yellow onions, new onions, and shallots, that can be interchanged in almost any recipe. Choose the type that suits your taste buds best to make your food delicious and healthy.

As stated earlier, you can use garlic and onions in soups, stews, casseroles, stir-fry, vegetables - keep the heat low, so you do not destroy the healthy properties. They are also great raw in salads, salad dressings and sandwiches. You can toss your steamed vegetables in garlic, onions, and olive oil - oh it smells and tastes so good! Make a Turkey Reuben sandwich with plenty of sauerkraut, chopped garlic and tomatoes to make a healthier sandwich. Prepare a delicious onion and garlic soup to ward off or help shorten the duration of colds and flu.

As noted, Garlic and Onions do some amazing things for the body that include:

- Killing viruses and bacteria
- Improving blood circulation
- May reduce risk of heart attack and stroke
- Killing fungus
- Reducing inflammation in the body

Health Tonic Formula

1. 8 Cloves of organic garlic
2. 6 ounces of Raw honey
3. 8 ounces of apple cider vinegar (unpasteurized)
4. Puree in a blender
5. Let sit in refrigerator for 3 days

6. Take one tablespoon per day

7. Make another batch before you finish this batch, and repeat daily

Make Garlic and Onions part of your daily meals, and your body will thank you.

CHAPTER 7:
YOUR ORAL HEALTH AFFECTS YOUR
OVERALL PHYSICAL HEALTH

Did you know that poor oral health can lead to cancer, diabetes, heart disease, stroke, high blood pressure, kidney failure, gum disease, pneumonia, and inflammation in the body? You may be shocked at what I tell you next. The way a dentist can identify if there is something wrong with a person's health is just by looking at their teeth and gums. If a person has red bleeding gums and cavities in their teeth, they most likely have heart disease, diabetes, a low-grade infection in their body, and very bad breath.

Untreated, these conditions are life threatening and can lead to heart attacks and kidney failure. In addition, if the person is under stress, their jaw muscles will be tight and their teeth will show indications that they routinely grind their teeth together while sleeping. This condition is known as bruxism, which leads to tooth damage, as well as, jaw and ear pain.

Also, doctors have known for years that type 2 diabetes has an increased incidence with evidence of periodontitis, or gum disease. Oftentimes, when infections in your mouth get bad enough, they can lead to low-grade inflammation throughout your body, which in turn wreaks havoc on your body's ability to process sugar, and can lead to heart disease.

As with diabetes, the connection between poor oral health and heart conditions has been recognized. According to research by the National Institutes of Health (NIH), small amounts of bacteria enter your bloodstream when you have bad teeth and diseased gums. The "bad" bacteria from an infected mouth may lodge itself inside blood vessels, ultimately causing dangerous blockages that lead to heart attacks and stroke.

As I mentioned, poor oral health can cause things to go horribly wrong in the body. The most obvious way poor oral health can affect you is that the individual will not be able to eat food properly. When your mouth hurts, it is difficult to chew food thoroughly resulting in poor digestion in the colon. Over time, this means the person's body will begin lacking the nutrients that it needs to stay healthy. Regular dental treatment and cleaning can prevent tooth decay, gum disease, and bad breath from occurring.

Also, an NIH study found that having a history of periodontal disease was associated with an increased risk of pancreatic and other cancers. According to the study, poor oral health could lead to systemic inflammation or increased levels of carcinogenic compounds produced in the infected mouth. Another viable theory about why gum disease may cause type 2 diabetes points to damage to the pancreas as well.

Healthy Mouth, Healthy Body

You already know that to avoid cavities and more serious dental problems, you must take good care of your teeth. Consistent brushing and daily flossing habits do more than just protect your oral health - they also help keep serious conditions at bay.

For improved oral health, here are some basic principles to follow:

- <u>Spend at least three minutes brushing your teeth 2 times a day, once in the morning and once in the evening before going to bed</u>. If needed, use a timer to ensure that you're spending enough time on your oral care routine.

- <u>Use floss at least once a day to clean between your teeth</u>.

- Buy American Dental Association (ADA) - approved dental cleaning tools and toothpaste. Motorized tooth brushes work very well.

The goal of regular home dental care is to combat the buildup of plaque in and around your teeth and gums, fight bad breath, tooth decay, and gum disease. Adults and children who neglect their teeth and who let plaque buildup often develop infections in the delicate tissue around their teeth, and can lead to tooth loss.

Good News

The good news is that by being diligent about your dental health care and getting regular dental checkups, you can prevent plaque from forming and even reverse early gum disease. A plaque-free mouth is a healthy mouth. Following good dental habits will decrease the probability of developing life-threatening diseases and allow you to enjoy a healthy disease-free life.

CHAPTER 8:
WHY SLEEP HELPS YOU AGE SLOWER AND KEEPS YOU HEALTHY

Have you ever had a deep refreshing night's sleep, and awaken feeling like a new person? There's a reason. It has been well documented that good sleeping habits will significantly enhance general wellbeing and extend your life. During sleep, your body regenerates from the rigors of the day. Quite a few functions occur during sleep. Let's explore what occurs.

First, your body detoxifies (removes harmful substances), which is extremely important for disease prevention and maintenance of good health. Primary to this function are the liver, kidney, and lungs.

The liver's main job is to filter the blood coming from the digestive tract, before passing it onto the rest of the body. In addition, the liver detoxifies the blood of chemicals and metabolizes drugs (i.e., changes these substances to a form that the body can use). As it works, the liver secretes bile that ends up back in the intestines. Bile is concentrated and stored in the gallbladder, and empties into the small intestine when needed for digestion. Bile helps in alkalinizing (i.e., balance the PH level of the body) the intestinal contents and plays a role in breaking down fat, helps with absorption, and digestion of fat. The liver also makes proteins important for blood clotting and other functions. Your liver detoxifies harmful substances in two steps. The first step uses enzymes and oxygen to burn toxins, especially fatty ones, so they are more water soluble, making them easier for the body to eliminate.

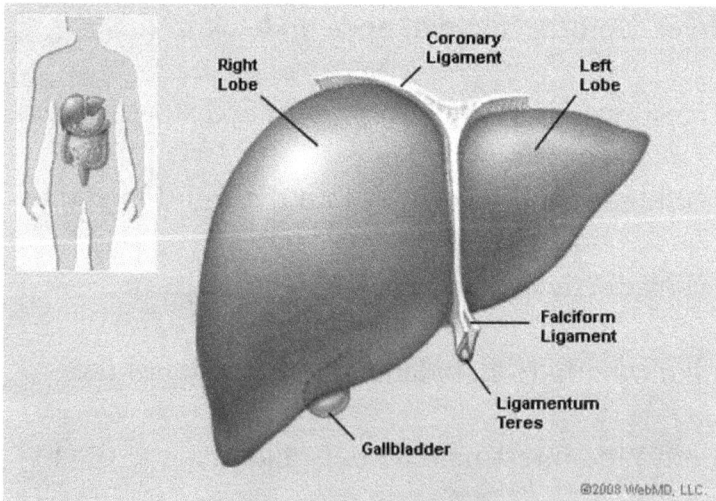

The kidneys detoxify the body by filtering about 120 to 150 quarts of blood a day to produce about 1 to 2 quarts of urine, composed of waste and excess fluid. The urine flows from the kidneys to the bladder. The bladder stores urine and remains relaxed until the bladder fills with urine. As the bladder fills to capacity, it signals the brain, so that you can find a toilet before you have a situation.

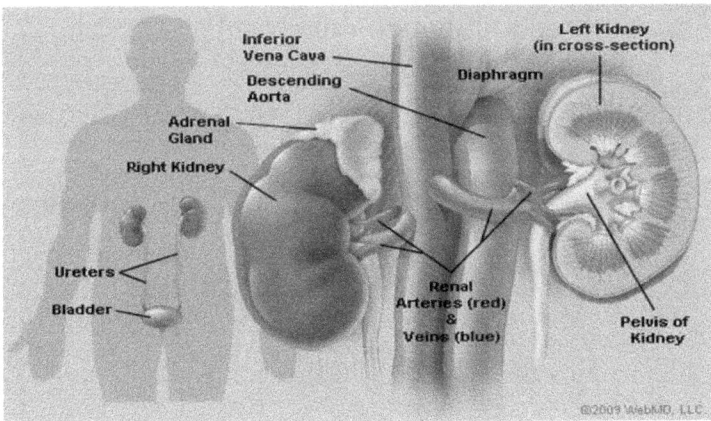

The lungs are another important component of the body's detoxification process. Let's explore how the lungs work. Breathing starts at the nose and mouth. You inhale air into your nose or mouth, and it travels down the back of your throat and into your windpipe, or trachea. Your trachea then divides into air passages called bronchial tubes.

For your lungs to perform their best, these airways need to be open during inhalation and exhalation, and free from swelling and excess or abnormal amounts of mucus. As the bronchial tubes pass through the lungs, they divide into smaller air passages called bronchioles. The bronchioles end in tiny balloon-like air sacs called alveoli -- your body has over 300 million. The alveoli are surrounded by a mesh of tiny blood vessels called capillaries. This is where oxygen from the inhaled air passes through the alveoli walls and into the blood.

After absorbing oxygen, the blood leaves the lungs and is carried to your heart, which pumps it through your body to provide oxygen to the cells of your tissues and organs.

As the cells use the oxygen, carbon dioxide is produced and absorbed into the blood. Your blood then carries the carbon dioxide back to your lungs, where it is removed from the body when you exhale.

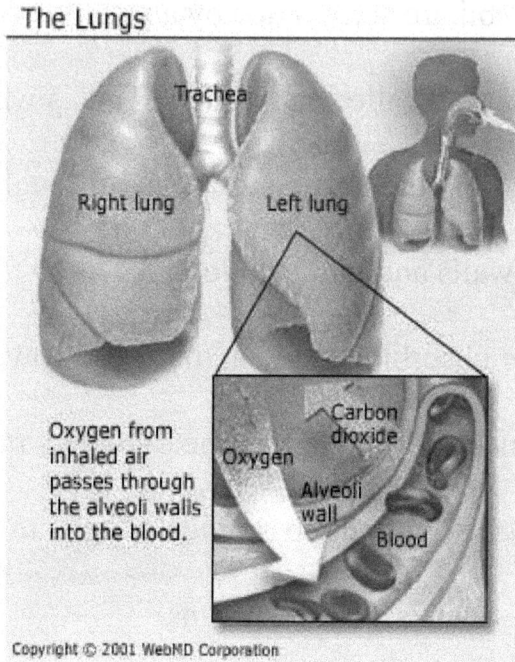

The Lungs

Trachea

Right lung

Left lung

Oxygen from inhaled air passes through the alveoli walls into the blood.

Oxygen

Carbon dioxide

Alveoli wall

Blood

Now that we've reviewed the vital organs involved with detoxification, let's get back to sleep. During sleep, the body produces important hormones, restores the immune system, executes waste elimination, and restores energy to all the cells in the body. These functions are key to slowing the process of aging, to increase your vitality and enhance brain function. During deep sleep, called REM (Rapid Eye Movement) sleep, your subconscious mind takes over in the form of dreaming, processing all the visual, audio, and tactile stimulation you experience over the course of the day. This process is important for mental health, as well as, enhancing brain function and allowing short-term memory to transfer to long-term memory – a process called synaptic development.

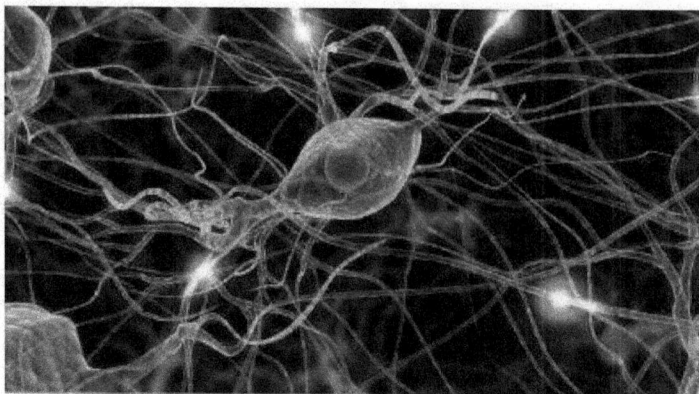

How much sleep do you need? As a rule of thumb, the average adult needs eight hours of sleep a day, plus or minus one hour. However, children need anywhere from 9 to 11 hours of sleep a day as they grow into adulthood.

People who don't get enough sleep often have poor physical and mental health, and have obvious physical and cognitive signs of aging.

Further, a lack of consistent good sleep could lead to illness and death.

On a final note, interesting enough, people who live to a healthy 100 or more get at least eight hours of sleep a night. Please note, good sleeping patterns are key to your physical and mental health, which has a direct relationship to a long healthy life.

CHAPTER 9:

HOW TO LIVE TO 100 AND BEYOND

NKJV Genesis. 6:3: The Creator said, "My Spirit shall not strive with man forever, because he also is flesh; nevertheless, his days shall be one hundred and twenty years."

What's the secret to live to 100 and beyond? Let's explore it.

Today, the world's most intriguing demographic is Generation C - those folks who are 100 years old and over. In the United States, the number of centenarians doubled in the 1980s and did so again in the 1990s. In fact, the total now exceeds 70,000, according to the U.S. Census Bureau. By 2050, according to midrange projections, there could be over 800,000 Americans who celebrate the century mark. Studies show the same trend in other industrialized countries as well. Moreover, demographers are now conducting a count of the number of *supercentenarians*, people age 110 and over to determine the size of that group.

The swelling population of people age 100 and over has given researchers an opportunity to answer some of the most fundamental questions about human health and longevity.

What does it take to live a long life? How much does diet, exercise, and other lifestyle factors matter compared with "good" genes? Perhaps most importantly, what is the quality of life among the very "old"? Does getting older inevitably mean getting sicker, or can people remain productive, social, and independent on their 100th birthday and beyond?

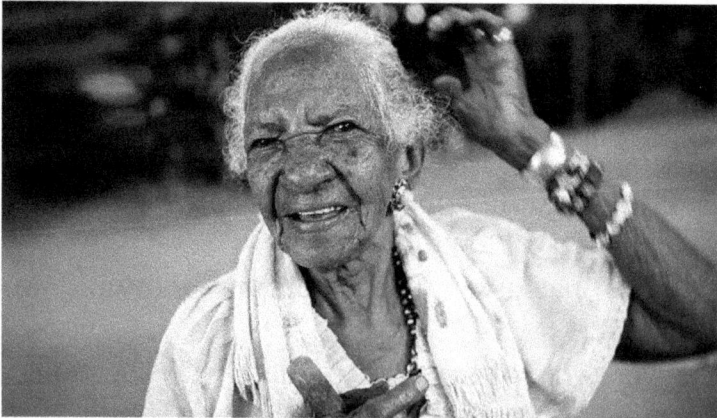

How Does Diet Play a Part?

One common thread in the long and healthy lives of people who live to be 100 plus is diet. Let's dig deeper into the healthy diet that leads to a long healthy life.

Most people who live to be 100 conform to diets that entail raw or lightly cooked vegetables and fruit that form the staple of their meals. The diet also includes healthy fats found in olive oil and salmon, along with a few saturated fats found in meat and dairy.

Olive Oil

A good number of centenarians consume extra virgin oil with most of the food they eat. They cook vegetables in it, dip bread into it, drizzle salad with it, use it in soups, and even drink a spoonful a day. Extra Virgin Olive oil is unrefined, so it retains all the healthy nutrients.

Olive oil is heart healthy and contains fat soluble vitamins A and E, which has been known to prevent cholesterol from oxidizing (i.e., damaging body cells and damaging arteries), as well as, raises the level of good HDL cholesterol, which pushes excess fat out of the bloodstream and out of the body via the stool. Olive oil may also have anticancer properties as well. It promotes cell health by enhancing cellular formation and cell membrane development. Research at Northwestern University in Chicago found that a substance in Olive oil called oleic acid significantly reduces the level of a cancer-causing gene called HER-2/neu, which is thought to be associated with breast cancer.

Olive oil also helps with digestion by triggering the gall bladder to release bile, purging undigested food, and lubricating the intestinal tract. In addition, Olive oil has antifungal properties that prevent candida (i.e., intestinal infection caused by fungus) overgrowth, and protects friendly intestinal flora

(bacteria). Olive oil also helps with circulation

to the erogenous areas of the body. Greeks have

a saying, "Eat butter and sleep tight, eat olive oil

and come alive at night". The healthy properties

of olive oil are best preserved in its raw state,

and is a key component in anti-aging.

Fruit and Vegetables

Fruit and vegetables are another key to

longevity. The longest living people eat five to

seven servings daily. They enjoy a variety of

fruit to include apples, blueberries, apricots,

lemons, watermelons, pineapples, peaches,

pears, oranges, bananas, grapes, cherries, melons, and papayas.

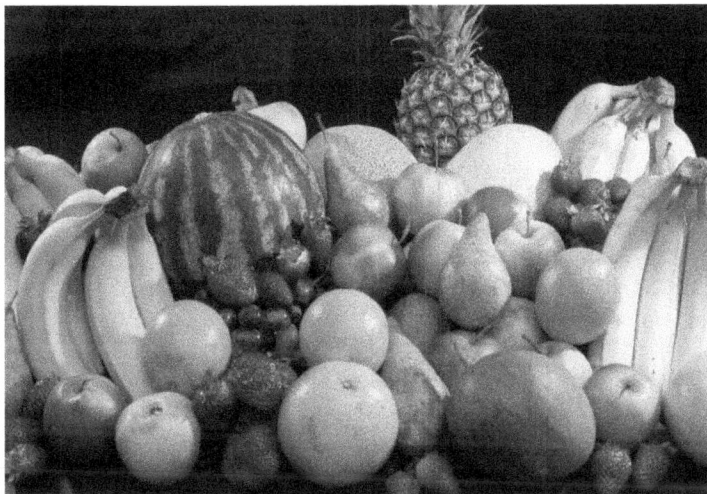

The long lived also eat plenty of servings of kale, collard greens, garlic, onions, broccoli, spinach, yams, sweet potatoes, brussel spouts, artichokes, eggplant, cabbage, green beans, seaweed, carrots, cauliflower, arugula, asparagus, fennel, lettuce, zucchini, celery, peas, chili peppers, mushrooms, and radish.

Unfortunately, most people don't eat enough raw antioxidant rich fruit and vegetables; however, the long lived clearly have the wisdom to eat those foods. One could say that the most common cause of aging is a vegetable and fruit deficiency.

People who live long understand that eating healthy doesn't have to be bland. They spice up food with garlic, onions, herbs, and spices. Herbs such as basil, oregano, thyme, parsley, and rosemary can be used in soups, casseroles, salads, and roasted vegetable dishes to enhance the flavor of food. These herbs also help with digestion, relives gas, balance healthy intestinal bacteria, and have antifungal properties.

Centenarian Studies

There are a dozen or so centenarian studies. A health-advice book that was published based on findings from a centenarian study in Okinawa, Japan, discovered that the average life expectancy of Japanese is 81.2 years, which is the highest in the world. In addition to Japan, there are active centenarian studies in Italy, Sweden, and Denmark. For the most part, results from these studies put to rest the myth that the oldest of the old are decrepit and dependent. Frail individuals die sooner, leaving a relatively robust group remaining alive. In fact, one of the rewards of living a long life is that, for the most part, the "extra" years are healthy years. Physical activity is a recurring theme - the people in these studies are walkers, bikers, and golfers. In Okinawa, centenarians do tai chi and karate. People who live to 100 and beyond exercise their brains, too, by reading, painting, and playing musical instruments. Some even continue to work, which allows them to remain physically and mentally active.

Good Genes

Traits that occur in families are not necessarily genetic. After all, families often share the same eating habits, activity levels, and other so-called environmental factors that influence health. Still, similarities within families are often a good clue of a strong genetic influence, and longevity does seem to run in some families. A New England Centenarian Study, for example, has found that its subjects were four times more likely to have a sibling who lived past age 90, than people with an average life span of 79 years. Based on that observation, the search is on for genetic attributes that run-in families.

The Gender Gap

Female centenarians outnumber males by a 9 to1 ratio. The longest documented life was that of a French woman, Jeanne Calment, who died in 1997 at the age of 122. Throughout most of the world, women, on average, live longer than men. Some researchers say it is estrogen that gives women the longevity edge. While other researchers theorize that menstruation and attributes related to childbirth better equip women to rid their bodies of toxins, which lead to adverse health conditions and death. Women also tend to be more social than men, and social connections are believed to be critical to weathering old age.

Men, however, who reach their 100th birthday are overall healthier than women around the same age. They are far less likely to have dementia or other serious medical problems. Thomas Perls, head of the New England Centenarian Study, calls these men "Aging Superstars."

Longevity statistics favoring women suggest that there may be some protective genes lurking on the X chromosome, the sex chromosome that women have two copies and men only one.

Another possibility is that genetics are relatively neutral with social activity favoring long life for women. Healthy odds-defying 100-year-old gentlemen hint of having healthy slow aging genes somewhere else in their genome.

Living to 100 is a blessing

What can you do to live a healthy productive life well into the 100's? The answer is easy, do what centenarians do.

If you aren't living a healthy lifestyle today, there may be hope. You can make choices that may help you catch up. There are lessons to be learned from the Do's and Don'ts of centenarians:

120

Do's:

- Eat a diet high in nutrients and moderate in calories, until you are 80% full

- Consume plenty of fresh fruit and vegetables without pesticides from local sources, if possible

- Eat fresh fish, such as salmon, sardines, and anchovies, at least three times a week

- Drink six (6) to eight (8) glasses of water daily

- Use olive oil regularly

- Eat whole grains rather than refined foods

- Eat vegetable protein, such as organic soy

- Drink alcohol in moderation, no more than three drinks per week

- Exercise daily

- Stay busy, but stress free

- Live in a loving manner and socialize regularly

Don't:

- Smoke

- Drink alcohol in excess

- Overeat

- Eat food high in sodium, or put too much salt on your food

- Overcook your food

- Eat white sugar or candy

- Eat processes foods, such as fast food, white bread, and too many sweets

- Live a risky or reckless life

- Drink 2 or more cups of coffee daily

People who live 100 plus years aren't doing anything mysterious. They're simply following the Creator's health commandments: eat a balanced diet comprised of vegetables, fruit, fiber; drink plenty of water daily; don't eat processed foods; don't smoke; don't drink alcohol in excess; don't ingest illegal drugs or substances; stay trim; get exercise daily; manage stress and avoid social isolation. May the Creator bless you as you live the centenarian lifestyle for a long healthy life full of vitality

AKNOWLEDGEMENTS

I first thank the creator for wisdom, understanding, health and strength. For without the creator, I am nothing. I also thank my mother Louise, who allowed me to experience life in such a way that I've evolved into the strong man that I am today. I acknowledge the memory of my sister Molly, who made a lasting impression on my life with her demonstration of love and kindness. Last, but not least, I thank my wife, Monique, whose love and support has allowed me to become a more empathic and caring man.

RECIPES

I include some healthy recipes for you to enjoy. Try eating healthy and balanced. Vary your diet by eating a range of healthy foods, instead of repeating the same meals from week to week. By eating healthy foods on a regular basis, you will receive the cumulative benefits over your lifetime. All the best as you Live the Way the Creator Intended.

Grilled Fish with Greens and Baked Sweet Potato

- 1 sweet potato
- 11 ounces or more of fish (e.g., cod, salmon, fresh tuna, mackerel, mahi mahi, rainbow trout, herring)
- Juice of 1 lemon
- 1 tablespoon of extra-virgin olive oil
- 5 ounces of spinach

1. Baked the sweet potato in oven at 375 degrees F for 40 minutes
2. Grill fish with a small amount of lemon and the olive oil for 5 to 10 minutes on each side, until cooked through medium well
3. Steam the spinach over boiling water for 4 minutes and serve with the fish and sweet potato. Serves 2 to 3.

Pasta with Roasted Red Peppers

- 4 red peppers
- 2 tablespoons of extra -virgin olive oil
- 1 clove of garlic, chopped
- Dash of sea salt
- 7 ounces of penne pasta

1. Bring 4 - 6 quarts of water to a rolling boil, add salt to taste.
2. Add penne pasta to boiling water, stirring occasionally for11 minutes. Remove from heat.
3. Grill the peppers with olive oil until browned all over, let cool for 20 minutes, then skin and remove insides
4. Toss the peppers in garlic, olive oil, and a small pinch of salt. Serves 2

Kale, Kidney, Cannellini, and Black Beans with Turkey Kielbasa

- 1 12-ounce package of turkey kielbasa
- Coarse salt to taste

- Red-pepper flakes to taste
- ¼ cup of extra-virgin olive oil
- 1 yellow onion
- 2 carrots. Sliced into ¼ inch rounds
- 4 garlic cloves, smashed
- 1 tsp. fennel seed
- 8 cups of low-sodium vegetable stock
- 1 can (15 oz.) Kidney beans
- 1 can (15 oz.) Cannellini beans
- 1 can (15 oz.) Black beans
- 1 bunch kale, trimmed and chopped
- Juice of 1 lemon

1. Season the turkey kielbasa with salt and pepper flakes to taste.

2. Preheat an 8-quart pot over medium-high heat, then add 2 tablespoons of the olive oil. Add the turkey kielbasa and cook without turning until seared on one side, about 3 minutes. Turn over, stirring occasionally until browned.

3. Add the onion, carrots, garlic, and fennel seeds and cook until the onions are translucent, about 8 minutes. Add the broth and bring it to a boil. Rinse and drain the

beans, then add the beans, reduce the heat to low, cover, and simmer about 40 minutes.

4. Add the kale and simmer uncovered, adding more broth if the stew looks too thick, until the ingredients are tender, about 30 minutes more. Stir in the remaining 2 tablespoons olive oil and the lemon juice, and season with more pepper flakes and salt. Serves 4 to 6

Vegetable Stir Fry

- 4 tablespoons extra virgin olive oil
- 2 teaspoons curry powder
- 1 teaspoon red chili flakes
- ½ teaspoon ground cinnamon
- 1 package (18 oz.) Asian stir fry vegetables
- 1 ½ cups of Jasmine rice
- 2 cups unsweetened coconut milk
- 2 tablespoons crème fraiche
- 2 tablespoons water
- 1 cup frozen mango chunks
- sea salt and fresh cracked black pepper, to taste

1. In a wok add curry, chili flakes and cinnamon. Stir to warm up spices, about one minute.

2. Add veggies; simmer over medium heat for about 10 min or until soft.

3. Pour 3 cups water into the saucepan and add light salt. Increase the heat to medium and let the rice come to a quick simmer. Reduce heat to low and let rice simmer lightly and sit uncovered until all the liquid is absorbed. Cover the rice and remove from heat and let sit for 15 mins.

4. Continue to stir fry for another 10 min.

5. Pour in coconut milk, fold in crème fraiche; add water and extra spices if desired.

6. Add mango and let mixture simmer for another 10 min.

7. Season with salt and pepper to taste.

8. Serve in a bowl over jasmine rice. Serves 4 to 6 people.

Black Bean Salad

- 16 ounce can of white corn, drained or 3 ears of corn cooked and cut from cob
- 3-4 tablespoons lime juice
- 2 tablespoons of olive oil
- 1 tablespoon red wine vinegar
- ½ teaspoon of salt
- ½ teaspoon pepper
- 2 large tomatoes (I used can diced tomatoes, drained)
- 1 can of black beans, drained
- 1 small purple onion (I used ¼ Vidalia onion)
- 1 avocado, peeled & chopped
- ¼ c cilantro chopped
- ½ jalapeno pepper, seeded and chopped (more if desired)

Combine all ingredients and chill. Serves 2 to 3 people

Blackened fish Sandwiches

- ¼ cup sweet paprika
- 2 tablespoons ground thyme
- 2 teaspoons onion powder
- 1 teaspoon garlic powder
- 1 teaspoon salt
- ¼ teaspoon ground red pepper
- 1 stick butter
- 4 10oz grouper or cod
- 4 Kaiser Buns split, buttered, and toasted
- Cilantro Lime Mayonnaise
- Mango Salsa

Combine first 6 ingredients in shallow dish. Melt

butter in another shallow dish. Dip fish in

melted butter then coat with seasoning mixture.

Brown 6-8 min in medium hot cast iron skillet.

Prepare in batches. Keep warm in oven until all

are cooked. Spread mayo over buns, place fish on bottom bun and top with mango salsa and cover with top half of bun. Serves 4

Cilantro Lime Mayo

- 1 cup mayonnaise
- ¼ cup chopped fresh cilantro
- 1 tablespoon fresh lime juice
- Mix ingredients, cover and chill

Mango Salsa

- 1 mango, peeled and diced
- 1 jalapeno seeded and diced
- 1 small orange pepper, seeded and diced
- ½ small red onions
- 1 clove garlic
- 1 teaspoon olive oil
- ¼ teaspoon salt
- Fresh lime juice- 1 tablespoons

- Combine all ingredients, coat, cover and chill

Tortellini soup

- 3 (14.5 ounce) cans vegetable broth
- 2 (9-ounce) packages refrigerated spinach tortellini (can also use cheese or mushroom)
- 1 (14.5- ounce can diced tomatoes with garlic and onion with juice
- 4 sliced green onions
- 2 cloves garlic, minced
- 1 teaspoon dried basil
- Freshly grated Parmesan cheese

1. Bring broth to a boil in a large pot over

   medium- heat.

2. Add tortellini, tomatoes, green onions, garlic,

   and basil.

3. Bring to boil. Reduce heat to low. Simmer 10 minutes. Serve 4 to 6

Roasted Cod with Fresh Tomato Sauce

- 2 pounds of fresh cod, skin on (substitute haddock, hake, or any white fish you like)
- 4 tbsp. of extra-virgin olive oil
- 12 ounces of ripe tomatoes
- 2 strips of pared orange rind
- 1 fresh thyme sprig
- 6 fresh basil leaves
- Ground black pepper
- Steam French green beans

1. Preheat oven to 450 degrees.
2. Roughly chop the tomatoes, skin on
3. Heat 1 tbsp. of olive oil in a pan, add tomatoes, orange rind, thyme, and basil and simmer for 5 minutes until tomatoes are juicy and soft. Remove from heat

4. Press tomatoes through a fine screen, and discard remains in screen. Pour tomato sauce into a small pan and heat gently.

5. Cut the cod into 4 pieces and season.

6. Steam green beans until cooked

7. Heat the remaining olive oil in a pan and fry the cod, skin side down, until skin is crisp. Place fish on a greased baking sheet, skin side up, and roast in oven for 6 to 8 minutes until cooked through.

8. Serve on top of the steamed green beans and pour fresh tomato sauce over cod. Serves 4

www.ingramcontent.com/pod-product-compliance
Lightning Source LLC
Chambersburg PA
CBHW071133280326
41935CB00010B/1214